Mastering Breathwork: A Quick Guide to Achieving Emotional and Physical Well-being

Violet Payne

Preface

Dear Reader,

Welcome to the world of breathwork—a journey of self-discovery, healing, and empowerment. I'm thrilled to share this adventure with you.

This book invites you to explore the transformative power of your breath, delving into its role in emotional stability, wellness, and personal growth.

As you read, reflect, and practice, know that you're part of a community seeking greater peace, clarity, and vitality. If you ever feel lost or unmotivated, start with the activities section. These exercises offer hands-on experience and immediate benefits, making it easy to engage with breathwork.

So, take a deep breath, and let's dive in—together.

With gratitude,

Violet

Table of Contents

Chapter 1: Introduction to Breathwork

Understanding the Role of Breath in Emotional Stability

Take a moment to notice your breath. Inhale deeply, exhale slowly. With each breath, you are not only supplying oxygen to your body but also engaging in a subtle dance with your emotions. It's a dance we often overlook, yet its impact on our emotional well-being is profound. In our fast-paced lives, it's easy to fall into the habit of shallow breathing, or even holding our breath altogether, especially during moments of stress or uncertainty. Yet, is this breath-holding truly beneficial, as some might claim? The answer is unequivocally no.

When we hold our breath in response to anxiety, depression, or tension, we unwittingly signal to our brain that we are in a state of alarm. This triggers a cascade of stress hormones, including cortisol and adrenaline, disrupting the delicate balance of our brain's functioning. Enter *breathwork*—a practice deeply intertwined with the concept of emotional stability. While the term may evoke images of yoga mats and meditation cushions, it encompasses far more than mere physical exercises. At its core, breathwork is about cultivating a sense of emotional equilibrium, harnessing the power of the breath to anchor ourselves amidst life's storms.

Unlike other forms of constant breathing exercises, such as yoga or meditation, breathwork offers a direct path to emotional stability without the need for specialized equipment or esoteric practices. It is a simple yet profound tool accessible to anyone, anywhere, at any time.

Differentiating between Breathwork and Regular Breathing

At first glance, breathwork may appear synonymous with the act of breathing itself. However, a closer examination reveals a fundamental distinction between the two. Regular breathing is an automatic, involuntary process driven by the body's physiological needs for oxygen and carbon dioxide exchange. It operates effortlessly, without conscious intervention, sustaining life with each inhalation and exhalation.

In contrast, breathwork is a deliberate, conscious engagement with the breath, imbued with intention and purpose. It transcends the realm of basic survival, encompassing a diverse array of techniques designed to optimize the breath for various therapeutic, spiritual, and emotional purposes.

While regular breathing serves as the foundation of our existence, breathwork invites us to explore the boundless potential of the breath as a tool for transformation and healing.

Why Breathwork is Essential for Overall Wellness

In today's fast-paced world, where stress and anxiety often reign supreme, the importance of cultivating emotional and physical well-being cannot be overstated. Herein lies the transformative power of breathwork. By harnessing the breath as a vehicle for self-exploration and self-regulation, breathwork offers a pathway to profound healing and holistic wellness. Unlike conventional approaches to health and wellness, which may focus primarily on external interventions or pharmaceutical solutions, breathwork offers a holistic, non-invasive means of addressing the root causes of imbalance within the body and mind. Through breathwork, individuals gain access to a powerful tool for managing stress, reducing anxiety, and enhancing overall resilience in the face of life's challenges.

Furthermore, breathwork serves as a gateway to deeper states of consciousness and spiritual exploration, facilitating profound shifts in perception and awareness. Whether through simple mindfulness practices or more elaborate pranayama techniques, breathwork invites us to reconnect with the innate wisdom of our bodies and cultivate a sense of harmony and alignment with the world around us. In the pages that follow, we will explore the myriad benefits of breathwork for overall wellness, delving into its transformative potential to foster emotional stability, enhance mental clarity, and promote vibrant health. Through understanding the unique role of breathwork in our lives, we embark on a journey of self-discovery and empowerment, harnessing the breath as a catalyst for profound healing and transformation.

We will touch on the following benefits of breathwork:

⇒ It helps in changing the worst mood and emotional instability.

⇒ Regular breathing exercises enhance emotional regulation, reduce anxiety, and boost confidence and emotional control

⇒ It assists in getting relief from anxiety and other nervous problems.

⇒ Helping in regulating blood pressure, it prevents cardiovascular disorders.

⇒ It boosts creativity and productivity.

Activity: Breath Awareness Exercise

Spend 5 minutes each day simply observing your breath without trying to change it. Notice the natural rhythm and how it feels in your body.

Chapter 2: The Fundamentals of Breathwork

Breathwork is a profound practice that encompasses both ancient wisdom and modern science, offering a pathway to inner transformation and holistic well-being. In this chapter, we delve into the fundamental principles of breathwork, exploring its multifaceted effects on our physical, emotional, and mental health. From the intimate connection between breath and emotions to the neurobiological mechanisms underlying breathwork practices, we uncover the essential elements that form the foundation of this transformative discipline.

Exploring the Connection between Breath and Emotions

Breath is not merely a passive physiological process but a dynamic reflection of our inner emotional landscape. When we experience joy, our breath may become light and expansive, effortlessly filling our lungs with each inhalation. Conversely, in moments of sadness or anxiety, our breath may become shallow and constricted, mirroring the tightness we feel in our chests. By tuning into these subtle shifts in our breathing patterns, we gain access to valuable insights into our emotional state.

Through breathwork practices such as conscious breathing and pranayama, we can consciously modulate our breath to influence our emotional experience. By deepening the breath and extending the exhalation, we can promote feelings of calmness and relaxation, soothing the nervous system and alleviating feelings of stress or anxiety. Conversely, by invigorating the breath with techniques like Kapalabhati (skull-shining breath), we can energize the body and uplift the spirits, fostering a sense of vitality and joy.

How Breathwork Affects the Brain and Stress Response

The breath serves as a potent regulator of both brain activity and the body's stress response system. Through intentional breathwork practices, we wield the power to influence the intricate dance between the autonomic nervous system and the brain, fostering profound changes in our physiological and psychological state.

Deep, diaphragmatic breathing serves as a catalyst for this transformation, stimulating the vagus nerve—a vital component of the parasympathetic nervous system. Activation of the vagus nerve triggers the body's "rest and digest" response, promoting relaxation and counteracting the physiological effects of stress. By engaging in diaphragmatic breathing, we tap into the body's innate capacity for resilience, enhancing our ability to navigate life's challenges with grace and equanimity.

Furthermore, breathwork harnesses the neuroplasticity of the brain, facilitating adaptive changes in neural pathways associated with stress regulation and emotional well-being. Through regular practice, breathwork cultivates a state of heightened awareness and presence, fostering a deep sense of connection with ourselves and the world around us.

Simple Techniques to Initiate Breathwork Practice

Embarking on a breathwork journey need not be intimidating; rather, it can be approached with simplicity and ease. By incorporating basic yet powerful techniques into our daily routine, we lay the foundation for a transformative breathwork practice that nurtures body, mind, and spirit.

Diaphragmatic breathing, also known as belly breathing, stands as a cornerstone of breathwork practice. By consciously engaging the diaphragm and fostering deep, rhythmic inhalations and exhalations, we promote relaxation and grounding, anchoring ourselves in the present moment.

This foundational technique sets the stage for deeper exploration into the realms of breathwork.

Box breathing offers another accessible entry point into the practice of breathwork. This technique, favored by athletes and military personnel alike, involves inhaling, holding, exhaling, and holding the breath in equal counts. By synchronizing breath with movement, we cultivate mental clarity and focus, fostering a sense of calm amidst the chaos of daily life. Box breathing serves as a bridge to the more advanced breathwork techniques we will explore in the following sections.

Breath awareness meditation invites us to simply observe the natural flow of the breath without judgment or manipulation. By cultivating present-moment awareness and inner stillness, we deepen our connection with the breath and unlock the transformative potential of breathwork in our lives. This practice prepares us for the nuanced exploration of breathwork techniques tailored to specific needs and intentions.

As we integrate these simple techniques into our daily lives, we pave the way for a profound journey of self-discovery and healing through the practice of breathwork. With each breath, we invite greater peace, clarity, and vitality into our being, awakening to the inherent wisdom of the breath and its transformative power to nurture body, mind, and spirit. In the following sections, we will delve into the techniques and benefits of nostril breathing, mantra breathing, belly breathing, and focused breathing, each offering unique pathways to inner peace and holistic well-being.

Activity: Emotional Connection Journal

Keep a journal for a week, noting how your breath changes with your emotions. Record instances of shallow breathing and deep breathing, and how they correlate with your feelings.

Chapter 3: Types of Breathwork Exercises

Breathwork encompasses a variety of techniques, each offering unique pathways to inner peace, emotional balance, and enhanced well-being. In this chapter, we will explore four fundamental types of breathwork exercises, each with its own set of techniques and benefits.

I. Belly Breathing: Connecting with the Body for Deep relaxation

Belly breathing, or diaphragmatic breathing, focuses on engaging the diaphragm to facilitate deep, rhythmic breaths. Unlike shallow chest breathing, which triggers the body's stress response, belly breathing activates the parasympathetic nervous system, promoting relaxation and reducing tension.

Here's how to practice belly breathing:

1. Find a comfortable seated position or lie down on your back.
2. Place one hand on your abdomen and the other on your chest.

3. Inhale deeply through your nose, allowing your abdomen to expand. Feel your hand rise as your belly expands.

4. Exhale slowly through your mouth or nose, gently contracting your abdominal muscles to expel the air. Feel your hand lower as your belly deflates.

5. Continue this deep, rhythmic breathing pattern for several minutes, focusing on the sensation of your breath.

Belly breathing promotes deep relaxation, alleviates anxiety, and enhances overall well-being by activating the parasympathetic nervous system.

II. Box Breathing: Cultivating Mental Clarity and Focus

Box breathing, or square breathing, is favored by athletes and military personnel for its ability to enhance mental clarity and focus.

Here's how to practice box breathing:

1. Find a comfortable seated position with your back straight and feet flat on the floor.

2. Inhale deeply through your nose for a count of four seconds.

3. Hold your breath for a count of four seconds.

4. Exhale slowly through your mouth or nose for a count of four seconds.

5. Hold your breath for a count of four seconds before beginning the next inhalation.

6. Repeat this cycle for several minutes, focusing on the rhythmic pattern of your breath.

Box breathing synchronizes breath with movement, creating a harmonious rhythm that promotes mental clarity, focus, and inner balance.

III. Nostril Breathing: Techniques and Benefits for Anxiety Relief

Nostril breathing, also known as alternate nostril breathing or Nadi Shodhana, is a potent breathwork technique rooted in ancient yogic practices. This practice involves the rhythmic alternation of breath between the left and right nostrils, facilitating the harmonization of prana (life force energy) throughout the body.

Here's how to practice nostril breathing:

1. Sit comfortably with your spine straight and shoulders relaxed.
2. Use your right thumb to close your right nostril and inhale deeply through your left nostril.
3. Close your left nostril with your ring finger, then release your thumb from your right nostril and exhale completely through the right nostril.
4. Inhale deeply through the right nostril, then close it with your right thumb and release your ring finger from the left nostril.
5. Exhale completely through the left nostril.
6. Continue this alternating pattern for several minutes.

Nostril breathing promotes deep relaxation, reduces anxiety, and enhances mental clarity and focus.

IV. Mantra Breathing: Harness the Power of Sound for Focus and Relaxation

Mantra breathing combines rhythmic breathing with the repetition of a sacred sound or phrase, known as a mantra. This practice offers a gateway to deep relaxation and heightened states of awareness.

The rhythmic cadence of the breath synchronized with the soothing resonance of the mantra creates a harmonious synergy that calms the mind and soothes the spirit. As practitioners immerse themselves in the gentle ebb and flow of breath and sound, they enter a state of profound tranquility, free from the distractions of the external world.

Here's how to practice mantra breathing:

1. Choose a mantra that resonates with you, such as "Om" or "peace."
2. Sit comfortably with your eyes closed and spine straight.
3. Inhale deeply through your nose, silently repeating your chosen mantra.
4. Exhale slowly through your mouth or nose, continuing to repeat the mantra with each breath.
5. Allow the sound of the mantra to anchor your awareness, guiding you into a state of deep relaxation and focus.

Mantra breathing reduces stress, enhances focus, and helps access higher states of consciousness and spiritual insight.

Activity: Practice Different Techniques

Try each type of breathwork exercise (belly breathing, box breathing, nostril breathing, and mantra breathing) for at least 5 minutes each day. Reflect on which technique resonates most with you.

Chapter 4: Integrating Breathwork into Daily Life

In the hustle and bustle of modern life, it's easy to overlook the profound impact that breathwork can have on our overall well-being. By integrating breathwork into our daily routines, we unlock the transformative power of the breath to cultivate inner peace, resilience, and vitality.

I.   Establishing a Breathwork Routine for Morning, Evening and Stressful Situations

Start and end your day with breathwork to set the tone for your overall well-being. In the morning, begin with a few minutes of deep, intentional breathing to center yourself and set positive intentions for the day. In the evening, unwind with calming breathwork practices like gentle belly breathing or soothing nostril breathing.

During stressful moments, turn to your breath. Techniques like box breathing or nostril breathing can activate the body's relaxation response and help regain a sense of calm and equilibrium. Remember, the breath is always available as a source of strength and support.

II.   Incorporating Breathwork into Existing Wellness Practices

Breathwork and mindfulness practices like yoga and meditation complement each other, enhancing overall benefits. In yoga, let your breath guide your movements and deepen your connection to the present moment. Incorporate specific breathwork techniques like ujjayi breath or kapalabhati to amplify the effects of your practice.

In meditation, use the breath as an anchor for the mind. Whether practicing focused breathing, loving-kindness meditation, or mindfulness of breath, each inhale and exhale can draw you deeper into the present moment, opening the door to tranquility and insight.

III.   Tips for Maintaining Consistency and Progress in Breathwork Practice

Consistency is key to reaping the full benefits of breathwork. Incorporate it into your daily habits and rituals. Use technology, journals, planners, and curated playlists on platforms like Spotify and YouTube to help you stick to a schedule.

Set realistic goals for your breathwork practice and monitor your progress. Celebrate your successes, no matter how small. Seek support from a community of like-minded individuals. Joining a breathwork class or online community can provide inspiration, encouragement, and guidance.

By integrating breathwork into your daily life with intention and consistency, you create space for profound healing, transformation, and self-discovery. Embrace the power of the breath as a guiding force for living with greater presence, resilience, and vitality.

Activity: Create a Breathwork Routine

Design a simple breathwork routine for your mornings and evenings. Start with 5-10 minutes and gradually increase the duration. Write down your routine and track your progress for two weeks.

Chapter 5: Transformative Benefits of Breathwork

Breathwork is more than just a wellness trend—it's a powerful tool that can profoundly impact various aspects of our lives. In this chapter, we'll delve into how breathwork can enhance emotional stability, boost confidence, manage anxiety, improve cardiovascular health, and increase creativity and productivity. By understanding these benefits, you'll gain insight into the comprehensive impact breathwork can have on your overall well-being.

I.   Enhancing Emotional Stability and Mood Regulation

Emotional stability is crucial for navigating life's ups and downs with resilience and grace. Breathwork offers effective techniques to regulate mood and cultivate emotional balance. Deep breathing exercises, such as diaphragmatic breathing and nostril breathing, activate the body's relaxation response, calming the mind and soothing turbulent emotions. By incorporating these practices into your daily routine, you can develop greater emotional resilience and respond to challenges with clarity and equanimity.

II. Overcoming Personality Challenges and Cultivating Confidence

Low self-esteem and personality challenges can significantly impact your quality of life. Breathwork provides a pathway to overcome these obstacles and build confidence from within. Practices like mindful breathing and positive affirmations promote self-awareness and self-compassion, empowering you to challenge negative thought patterns and embrace your true self. Over time, breathwork helps cultivate a strong sense of confidence and self-worth, positively influencing every aspect of your life.

III. Managing Anxiety and Nervous System Disorders

Anxiety and nervous system disorders can be debilitating, affecting both mental and physical well-being. Breathwork offers effective strategies for managing these conditions and restoring a sense of calm and balance. Techniques like box breathing, where inhalation, retention, and exhalation are equal in duration, help regulate the autonomic nervous system and reduce physiological symptoms of anxiety. Progressive muscle relaxation combined with deep breathing further enhances relaxation and alleviates tension. By practicing these techniques consistently, you can develop greater resilience to stress and anxiety, leading to improved overall well-being.

IV.   Promoting Cardiovascular Health and Blood Pressure Regulation

The health of our cardiovascular system is vital for longevity and vitality. Breathwork plays a crucial role in supporting cardiovascular health and regulating blood pressure. Deep breathing exercises, such as belly breathing and heart-focused breathing, improve circulation, reduce inflammation, and promote relaxation. These practices also help regulate blood pressure by activating the body's parasympathetic nervous system, which counteracts the stress response. By integrating breathwork into your daily routine, you can optimize the health of your heart and vascular system, reducing the risk of cardiovascular disease and enhancing overall vitality.

V. Boosting Creativity, Productivity and Overall Well-Being through Breathwork

Creativity and productivity thrive in an environment of relaxation and mental clarity. Breathwork provides a natural pathway to unlock your creative potential and enhance productivity. By quieting the mind and reducing stress, breathwork creates the ideal conditions for inspiration to flow freely. Techniques like rhythmic breathing and alternate nostril breathing improve focus, concentration, and cognitive function, leading to increased productivity and efficiency. Moreover, regular breathwork practice boosts overall well-being by reducing stress levels, improving sleep quality, and fostering a greater sense of contentment and fulfillment in life.

In conclusion, breathwork is a multifaceted practice with profound benefits for emotional, mental, and physical health. By incorporating breathwork into your daily life, you can cultivate greater emotional stability, confidence, and resilience, while also improving cardiovascular health, managing anxiety, and enhancing creativity and productivity. With dedication and consistency, breathwork has the power to transform every aspect of your life, leading to greater health, happiness, and fulfillment.

Activity: Breathwork for Specific Benefits

Choose one of the benefits discussed (e.g., managing anxiety, boosting creativity) and practice a related breathwork technique daily. Record any changes or improvements you notice over a week.

Chapter 6: The Path Forward with Breathwork

As we reach the final chapter, it's time to reflect on the journey of self-discovery and healing that breathwork has taken us on. We've explored its transformative power and the profound impact it can have on our physical, emotional, and mental well-being. In this chapter, we'll reinforce the importance of breathwork as a lifelong tool for wellness, celebrate your progress, and encourage you to continue embracing breathwork as a means to achieve emotional stability and holistic well-being.

I.   Reflecting on Personal Experiences and Progress

As we look back on our breathwork journey, it's essential to take stock of our personal experiences and the progress we've made. Whether we've experienced moments of profound insight, encountered challenges, or witnessed subtle shifts in our emotional and mental well-being, each step of our breathwork practice has been a valuable part of our growth and evolution.

- **Acknowledge Moments of Transformation:** Reflect on the moments of transformation and breakthroughs you've experienced during your breathwork practice. Consider the emotions, sensations, and insights that have arisen during your sessions, and how they have impacted your life outside of your practice.

- **Embrace Challenges and Growth Opportunities:** Acknowledge the challenges you've faced on your breathwork journey and the valuable lessons they've taught you. From moments of resistance to periods of discomfort, each challenge has presented an opportunity for growth, resilience, and self-discovery.

- **Celebrate Progress and Milestones:** Take a moment to celebrate the progress you've made in your breathwork practice, no matter how small or seemingly insignificant. Celebrate the moments of consistency, the breakthroughs in awareness, and the newfound sense of peace and clarity that breathwork has brought into your life.

II.   The Importance of Breathwork as a Lifelong Tool for Wellness

Breathwork is not just a temporary practice but a lifelong tool for self-awareness, resilience, and vitality. Its benefits extend beyond immediate relaxation, supporting long-term well-being on physical, emotional, and spiritual levels.

- **Cultivating Self-Awareness and Mindfulness:**
Breathwork serves as a powerful tool for cultivating self-awareness and mindfulness, allowing us to connect more deeply with ourselves and the present moment. By tuning into the breath, we learn to observe our thoughts, emotions, and sensations with curiosity and compassion, fostering greater insight and clarity.

- **Nurturing Emotional and Mental Well-Being:**
Breathwork provides a safe and supportive space to explore and process our emotions, helping us release pent-up tension, stress, and anxiety. Through regular practice, we cultivate greater emotional resilience, allowing us to navigate life's challenges with grace and ease.

- **Supporting Physical Health and Vitality:**
The benefits of breathwork extend beyond emotional and mental well-being, encompassing physical health and vitality as well. By promoting relaxation, reducing stress, and improving respiratory function, breathwork enhances our overall health and vitality, supporting longevity and well-being.

III.   Embrace the Adventure: Encouraging Exploration of Breathwork

As our breathwork journey draws to a close, let's ignite the spark of adventure within us and dive into the endless possibilities that lie ahead. Rather than seeing breathwork as a mere practice, let's embrace it as an odyssey—an ongoing quest of self-discovery, empowerment, and holistic flourishing.

- **Embrace Curiosity and Discovery:**
  Approach your breathwork practice with the curiosity of an explorer and the wonder of a child. Each breath becomes a gateway to new insights, revelations, and experiences. Embrace the unknown with an open heart and mind, ready to uncover the treasures hidden within.

- **Celebrate the Journey and Destination:**
  Infuse your breathwork practice with a sense of playfulness and creativity. Experiment with different techniques, rhythms, and modalities, trusting your intuition to guide you. From ancient yogic traditions to innovative modern approaches, let your imagination soar as you chart your unique course.

- **Embrace Community and Connection:**
  Seek support and camaraderie as you continue your breathwork adventure. Join a breathwork community, attend workshops and retreats, or connect with fellow

practitioners online. Remember that you're part of a vast network of kindred spirits, all journeying towards healing and transformation. Share your experiences, learn from others, and offer encouragement along the way.

IV.   Embodying the Breath: Living with Presence and Purpose

Let's now integrate the essence of breathwork into our daily lives, infusing each moment with presence, intention, and gratitude. Allow the insights gleaned from our practice to permeate our interactions, relationships, and endeavors, enriching every aspect of our existence with the transformative power of the breath.

- **Living with Presence:**
  As you continue your breathwork journey, strive to live each moment with presence and mindfulness. Let the practice of conscious breathing guide you through the complexities of daily life, helping you stay grounded and centered.

- **Cultivating Intention:**
  Approach each breathwork session and each day with clear intentions. Whether it's cultivating inner peace,

enhancing emotional resilience, or improving physical health, let your goals guide your practice and your actions.

- **Fostering Gratitude:**
  Embrace a mindset of gratitude for the breath and its transformative power. Appreciate the small victories and moments of clarity that come with your practice, and let gratitude enhance your overall sense of well-being.

Activity: Personal Reflection and Goal Setting

Reflect on your breathwork journey so far. Write about your experiences, challenges, and progress. Set specific goals for how you want to continue incorporating breathwork into your life.

Additional Activities to Consider

Guided Meditation Recordings: Check out guided breathwork meditations on popular platforms like YouTube, Healthy Minds, Insight Timer, and Calm. Search for specific techniques like "diaphragmatic breathing," "box breathing," "alternate nostril breathing," or "mantra breathing" to find sessions that fit your needs.

Partner Exercises: Try practicing breathwork with a partner or in a group to see how shared breathwork can enhance your experience.

Visualization and Breathwork: Combine visualization with breathwork. As you breathe deeply, imagine calmness entering your body with each inhale and stress leaving with each exhale.

Track Your Progress: Use online resources to find printable charts or templates for tracking your breathwork practice. Alternatively, you can start easily by using the notes app on your phone to record your sessions and note any changes in your emotional and physical well-being. Search for "breathwork practice tracker" or "well-being journal template" to find helpful tools that suit your needs.

Mindful Movement: Pair breathwork with gentle movements like yoga or tai chi. Try simple routines or poses that complement your breathwork practice.

As you embark on this journey as a new breathwork practitioner, remember that every breath is an opportunity for growth and healing. Stay curious, stay committed, and most importantly, be kind to yourself. Breathwork is a personal journey that unfolds uniquely for everyone. Celebrate your progress, no matter how small, and trust that each breath you take brings you closer to greater health, happiness, and fulfillment.

Take a moment to notice your breath—may your journey be filled with discovery, transformation, and peace.

www.ingramcontent.com/pod-product-compliance
Lightning Source LLC
Chambersburg PA
CBHW051721250726
48653CB00008B/3136